# WEIGHT WARRIORS

## CONFRONTING THE FAT EPIDEMIC, MOBILIZING AGAINST A SOCIETAL CRISIS

Alfonso Borello

Villaggio Publishing Ltd

# CONTENTS

# INTRODUCTION: A CALL TO ACTION

Picture this: you're walking down the street, and at every turn, you see something that breaks your heart – obese children. It's not just a few; it's everywhere. The sadness and disbelief hit you like a ton of bricks. How did we get here? How did we let it get this bad?

But this isn't just about feeling sad. It's about recognizing that we have a problem—a big problem—and it's time to do something about it. We're not talking about pointing fingers or blaming anyone. We're talking about taking action, about standing up and saying, "Enough is enough."

Because here's the thing: every parent has a responsibility—a moral obligation—to protect their child's health. It's not just about feeding them or keeping them safe; it's about ensuring they have the best chance at a happy, healthy life.

So, why are we seeing so many obese kids? It's not just because they're eating too much or not exercising enough. Sure, those things play a part, but there's more to it than that. We're up against a powerful enemy: the fast-food industry.

These guys are making a killing—literally—off of our kids' health. They're selling us greasy, unhealthy food, and they're making a fortune doing it. But at what cost? Our children's well-being, that's what.

We can't sit back and let this happen. We can't keep turning a blind eye while our kids suffer. It's time to stand up and fight back. And that's exactly what this book is about.

We're not here to make a profit or to point fingers. We're here to amplify the message, to spread the word, and to inspire action. We're here to shine a light on the truth and to demand change.

So, if you're reading this, know that you're not alone. We're in this together, and together, we can make a difference. It's time to Weight Warriors against the fat epidemic, and it starts now. Are you with us?

# CHAPTER 1: THE ALARMING RISE OF CHILDHOOD OBESITY

In recent years, there has been a troubling trend that cannot be ignored: the alarming rise of childhood obesity. No longer is it a distant concern relegated to medical journals; it's a reality staring us in the face every day, on every street corner, in every community.

The statistics paint a stark picture: rates of childhood obesity have more than tripled since the 1970s, with nearly one in five children and adolescents now classified as obese. This isn't just about carrying a few extra pounds; it's a serious health issue with far-reaching consequences.

Childhood obesity can cast a long shadow over a child's well-being, impacting them not just in the distant future but right now. Excess weight can disrupt sleep, leading to a condition called sleep apnea where breathing becomes erratic at night. This translates into daytime fatigue, making it hard to concentrate in school and participate fully in life. Carrying extra pounds also puts a strain on young muscles and joints, causing aches and pains especially in weight-bearing areas like knees, hips, and the back. This discomfort can become a barrier to physical activity, creating a frustrating cycle where limited movement leads to further weight gain and more aches.

The impact goes beyond the physical. Children with obesity are more susceptible to emotional distress. Teasing and bullying from peers can lead to feelings of isolation, depression, and low self-esteem. The pressure to conform to unrealistic body image standards adds another layer of difficulty. Negative body image and even eating disorders can develop, further affecting a child's mental and emotional health. Social stigma surrounding obesity can make them feel embarrassed and withdrawn, limiting their ability to connect with others and enjoy social activities.

But perhaps most concerning is the fact that childhood obesity often tracks into adulthood. A child who is obese is more likely to remain obese as an adult, compounding the health risks and placing further strain on healthcare systems already struggling to cope with the burden of chronic disease.

So, how did we get here? There are multiple factors at play, including changes in diet, lack of physical activity, and environmental influences. The rise of processed and fast food, coupled with sedentary lifestyles and increased screen time, has created a perfect storm for the obesity epidemic to flourish.

But here's the thing: we can't afford to sit back and watch this unfold. We can't accept childhood obesity as the new normal. It's time to take action—to confront the root causes of the problem and to work together to create a healthier future for our children.

In the chapters that follow, we'll delve deeper into the factors driving the rise of childhood obesity and explore strategies for combatting this growing epidemic. Together, we can make a difference. It's time to take a stand and fight back against childhood obesity.

# CHAPTER 2: THE MORAL IMPERATIVE OF PARENTAL RESPONSIBILITY

We, as parents, hold a sacred trust – to nurture, protect, and guide our children towards a vibrant future brimming with possibilities. At the heart of this responsibility lies safeguarding their health and well-being. After all, without a healthy foundation, all other aspirations become distant echoes.

Yet, as the tide of childhood obesity rises, a stark reality confronts us: we are failing in this sacred duty. Every day, more and more children succumb to a preventable, avoidable condition – one that casts a long shadow, not just on their physical health, but on their very future.

What does parental responsibility truly mean in the face of this crisis? It transcends the mere provision of food and shelter. It demands instilling healthy habits, embodying positive behaviors, and prioritizing our children's long-term well-being above all else.

It necessitates a brutal self-examination. We must acknowledge the impact our choices have on our children's health and be resolute in making changes, however difficult. It means resisting the siren call of fast-food convenience and processed snacks, and embracing the joys of home-cooked meals crafted from fresh, nourishing ingredients.

But nourishment goes beyond just the physical. It's about fostering a healthy relationship with food. We must guide our children to listen to their bodies, cultivate mindful eating habits, and embrace a balanced diet that satiates both body and spirit.

The road of parenthood is rarely smooth, and missteps are inevitable. However, when it comes to our children's health, there's no room for indifference. We must be willing to become students ourselves – to seek knowledge, gather support, and tirelessly strive to ensure our children grow strong, happy, and healthy.

In the following chapters, we'll delve into practical strategies for nurturing healthy eating habits and fostering active lifestyles within the family. We'll explore the power of leading by example, setting clear boundaries, and cultivating a positive food environment in our homes. Together, we can rise to the challenge of parental responsibility, creating a shield against the growing threat of childhood obesity.

The fight against childhood obesity is not one we can afford to lose. By acknowledging the moral imperative of parental responsibility, equipping ourselves with knowledge, and committing to consistent action, we can collectively rise to this challenge and ensure our children inherit a future where health and happiness are not aspirations, but a lived reality.

# CHAPTER 3: THE FAST-FOOD TRAP: PROFITING FROM POOR HEALTH

The ubiquitous presence of fast-food chains in our society, especially in the realm of children's experiences, masks a sinister reality. Beneath the alluring aroma of greasy fries and the sugary allure of sodas lies a meticulously engineered "trap" that places corporate profits above the well-being of consumers.

Fast-food entities have permeated every nook and cranny of our existence, luring us with the promise of effortless indulgence through convenient drive-thrus and the festive ambiance of themed playgrounds. These establishments have become synonymous with celebration and childhood bliss, eagerly embraced by parents seeking a respite from the demands of daily life.

However, this façade of convenience and enjoyment conceals a disturbing truth. Fast-food companies have meticulously constructed a marketing strategy that exploits the vulnerabilities of children and their parents. Mascots with endearing personalities and vibrant packaging create an illusion of wholesome entertainment, distracting from the nutritional deficiencies lurking beneath the delectable exterior.

Through relentless advertising campaigns, fast-food chains

have embedded their products deeply into our cultural consciousness, shaping our perceptions of what constitutes a "normal" meal. Their omnipresence has gradually eroded our understanding of healthy eating habits, making us more susceptible to the allure of their calorie-dense, nutrient-poor offerings.

The fast-food industry has become a formidable force in shaping our dietary choices, contributing to a public health crisis of obesity, chronic diseases, and diminished overall well-being. By prioritizing their bottom line over the health of individuals, fast-food companies have created a pervasive trap that threatens the well-being of future generations.

## Covid-19: a wake-up call for poor health

The COVID-19 pandemic has served as a stark wake-up call, shining a harsh spotlight on the dire consequences of poor health and destructive eating habits. Individuals with compromised immune systems, often weakened by years of unhealthy diets, found themselves particularly vulnerable to the virus. Bacterial infections that were once easily treated with antibiotics now posed a serious threat due to the emergence of antibiotic-resistant strains.

COVID-19 has exposed the fragility of our health infrastructure and the urgent need to address long-standing issues of dietary neglect. The fast-food industry's relentless pursuit of profit has contributed significantly to these health disparities, highlighting the need for systemic changes to prioritize public health over corporate interests.

As we grapple with the aftermath of the pandemic, it's become abundantly clear that our health is our greatest asset—and yet, it's one that we've too often taken for granted. We've allowed ourselves to be seduced by the convenience and affordability of fast food, sacrificing our well-being on the altar of expediency.

But the price we've paid has been steep. The toll of obesity, diabetes, and other diet-related diseases has exacted a heavy burden on individuals, families, and society as a whole. And now, in the wake of COVID-19, we're paying the price in lives lost, families shattered, and economies crippled.

It's time to break free from the fast-food trap and reclaim our health. It's time to reject the false promises of convenience and cheap thrills.

# CHAPTER 4: THE HIGH COST OF GREASY FARE: HEALTH IMPLICATIONS

Greasy fare may seem like a tempting indulgence in the moment—a guilty pleasure that promises instant gratification and satisfaction. But make no mistake: the true cost of consuming these greasy, unhealthy foods extends far beyond the immediate pleasure it provides. In this chapter, we will explore the profound health implications of indulging in greasy fare, shedding light on the toll it takes on our bodies and our well-being.

From heart disease to type 2 diabetes, the health risks associated with a diet high in greasy fare are well-documented and deeply concerning. These foods are often laden with saturated fats, trans fats, and cholesterol, all of which contribute to the buildup of plaque in the arteries, leading to atherosclerosis and an increased risk of heart attack and stroke.

But it's not just our cardiovascular health that suffers. Greasy fare is also a major contributor to obesity, a condition that has reached epidemic proportions in many parts of the world. Excess body weight not only places strain on the joints and organs but also increases the risk of developing a host of other chronic diseases, including type 2 diabetes, certain cancers, and fatty liver disease.

Moreover, greasy fare is often devoid of essential nutrients, such as vitamins, minerals, and fiber, leaving us feeling sluggish, lethargic, and unsatisfied. This can lead to overeating and further exacerbate the cycle of poor nutrition and weight gain.

But perhaps most concerning is the impact of greasy fare on our mental and emotional well-being. Studies have shown that a diet high in unhealthy fats and processed foods is associated with an increased risk of depression, anxiety, and other mood disorders. These foods may provide temporary comfort and pleasure, but in the long run, they leave us feeling drained, irritable, and emotionally unstable.

## Ah, emotionally unstable?

In light of these sobering realities, it's clear that we cannot continue to turn a blind eye to the high cost of greasy fare. Beyond its physical toll, the emotional and psychological consequences of consuming such foods are equally concerning.

When we rely on greasy fare as a source of comfort or escape, we may experience a temporary surge of pleasure or satisfaction. However, this fleeting sense of contentment is often followed by a crash—a wave of guilt, shame, and regret that washes over us, leaving us feeling emotionally drained and unstable.

Indeed the rollercoaster of highs and lows induced by greasy fare can wreak havoc on our mood and mental well-being. The spikes and crashes in blood sugar levels caused by sugary, processed foods can lead to irritability, mood swings, and difficulty concentrating. Meanwhile, the inflammatory response triggered by consuming high-fat, greasy foods can exacerbate feelings of anxiety and depression, leaving us feeling overwhelmed and emotionally fragile.

In the long term, relying on greasy fare as a coping mechanism can perpetuate a vicious cycle of emotional instability and poor dietary choices. We may turn to these foods in times of stress or sadness, seeking solace in their familiar embrace. Yet, far from providing comfort, they only serve to deepen our distress, leaving us trapped in a cycle of emotional turmoil and unhealthy habits.

## *Not convinced?*

When we consistently indulge in destructive eating habits, such as consuming greasy fare high in unhealthy fats, sugars, and processed ingredients, it can have detrimental effects not only on our physical health but also on our mental and emotional well-being.

One significant consequence of such eating habits is irritability. The rapid spikes and crashes in blood sugar levels caused by sugary and processed foods can lead to fluctuations in mood, leaving us feeling irritable, anxious, and easily agitated. These mood swings can disrupt our interactions with others, strain relationships, and impair our ability to cope with stressors effectively.

Indeed, poor dietary choices can also impact cognitive function and performance. Research suggests that diets high in greasy, unhealthy foods are associated with cognitive decline, impaired memory, and reduced mental clarity. When we fuel our bodies with nutrient-poor foods, we deprive our brains of the essential nutrients needed for optimal function, leading to sluggishness, brain fog, and poor concentration.

As a result, we may find ourselves struggling to focus on tasks, make decisions, or retain information. Our productivity may suffer, and we may experience a decline in overall performance at work, school, or in our daily activities. This can further contribute to feelings of frustration, inadequacy, and low self-esteem, creating a vicious cycle of emotional distress and poor performance.

Yes, the negative effects of destructive eating habits extend beyond our individual well-being to impact our broader social and professional interactions. Irritability and poor performance can strain relationships with coworkers, friends, and family members, leading to conflicts and misunderstandings. In professional settings, diminished productivity and cognitive function may jeopardize job performance and career advancement opportunities.

In essence, destructive eating habits not only compromise our physical health but also undermine our emotional stability and cognitive function, impairing our ability to navigate life's challenges effectively. Recognizing the link between diet and mood, and taking steps to prioritize nutritious, whole foods can help us regain control over our emotional well-being and optimize our performance in all aspects of life.

## *Navigating emotional eating: understanding affect regulation in destructive eating habits*

In the context of destructive eating habits, affect regulation refers to the process by which individuals use food as a means of managing or regulating their emotions. When faced with challenging or distressing feelings, such as stress, sadness, anxiety, or boredom, some individuals may turn to food as a way to cope or alleviate their discomfort.

For many people, food provides more than just sustenance; it offers a source of comfort, pleasure, and distraction from unpleasant emotions. Consuming high-fat, sugary foods can trigger the release of neurotransmitters, such as dopamine, in the brain, which produce feelings of pleasure and reward. This can create a temporary sense of relief or satisfaction, helping individuals to temporarily escape or numb their emotional pain.

However, relying on food as a primary means of affect regulation can lead to a pattern of maladaptive coping and contribute to the development of destructive eating habits. Over time, this behavior can become ingrained and habitual, making it difficult to break free from the cycle of emotional eating.

We must also stress that using food as a distraction from difficult emotions can prevent individuals from addressing the underlying issues contributing to their distress. Instead of confronting and processing their feelings in a healthy and constructive manner, they may continue to suppress or avoid them, perpetuating a cycle of emotional avoidance and overeating.

In addition, the temporary relief provided by food is often followed by feelings of guilt, shame, and regret, further exacerbating negative emotions and reinforcing the cycle of emotional eating. This can lead to a vicious cycle of emotional instability and destructive eating habits, which can have serious consequences for physical health, emotional well-being, and overall quality of life.

To break free from the cycle of emotional eating and destructive eating habits, it is important for individuals to develop alternative strategies for affect regulation that are healthier and more sustainable. This may involve learning and practicing healthy coping skills, such as mindfulness, relaxation techniques, journaling, or seeking support from friends, family, or mental health professionals.

By addressing the underlying emotions and learning to regulate them in a more adaptive manner, individuals can reduce their reliance on food as a coping mechanism and cultivate a healthier relationship with food and their emotions. This can lead to improved emotional well-being, better self-care practices, and a greater sense of control over one's eating habits and overall health.

# CHAPTER 5: MUTATION: UNRAVELING THE GENETIC AND ENVIRONMENTAL FACTORS

Obesity is not solely a matter of personal choice or willpower; rather, it is a complex interplay of genetic and environmental factors that shape our susceptibility to weight gain and influence our body's response to diet and exercise. In this chapter, we delve into the intricate relationship between genetics and the environment, exploring how these factors interact to predispose individuals to obesity and shape the course of the obesity epidemic.

Genetic factors play a significant role in determining an individual's predisposition to obesity. Research has identified numerous genes associated with obesity, each contributing in its own way to the regulation of appetite, metabolism, and fat storage. These genetic variations can influence factors such as hunger and satiety signals, energy expenditure, and the body's ability to process and store nutrients. Individuals who inherit certain genetic variants may be more susceptible to weight gain in environments where calorie-dense, high-fat foods are abundant and physical activity is limited.

However, genetics alone do not determine our fate. Environmental factors also play a crucial role in shaping our body composition and overall health. Our surroundings—such as our home, school, workplace, and community—can either support or hinder healthy behaviors, influencing our dietary choices, physical activity levels, and access to nutritious foods. In environments where unhealthy foods are cheap, convenient, and heavily marketed, and opportunities for physical activity are limited, individuals are more likely to succumb to obesity-promoting behaviors.

Unquestionably, the interaction between genetics and the environment is dynamic and bidirectional. Environmental factors can influence gene expression, altering the way our genes function and predisposing us to certain health outcomes. Conversely, genetic factors can influence our response to the environment, shaping our susceptibility to weight gain and metabolic disorders in different contexts.

In light of these complex interactions, addressing the obesity epidemic requires a multifaceted approach that addresses both genetic and environmental factors. This includes implementing policies and interventions that promote healthy behaviors, such as improving access to nutritious foods, creating safe and walkable environments, and providing education and support for lifestyle modifications.

By unraveling the genetic and environmental factors contributing to obesity, we can gain a deeper understanding of the underlying mechanisms driving the epidemic and develop more targeted and effective strategies for prevention and treatment. Together, we can empower individuals to overcome genetic predispositions and environmental barriers and achieve lasting improvements in their health and well-being.

## *A bit of science*

Mutation, the alteration of a genetic sequence, is a fundamental process that drives evolution and contributes to human health and disease. Understanding the causes and consequences of mutations is essential for advancing medical research and public health.

Genetic mutations can be inherited from parents, passed down through the germline (eggs and sperm), or occur during an individual's lifetime in non-germline cells. These mutations can lead to genetic disorders, such as sickle cell anemia, cystic fibrosis, and Huntington's disease, or increase the risk of cancer.

Environmental factors, such as radiation, chemicals, oxidative stress, and transposable elements, can also cause mutations by damaging DNA. These factors can increase mutation rates and contribute to the development of diseases like cancer.

Mutations come in various forms, including single nucleotide variants (SNVs), insertions and deletions (Indels), and copy number variations (CNVs). They can have significant effects on gene function, leading to changes in protein structure, gene expression, and cellular processes.

Advances in genome sequencing and gene-editing technologies, such as CRISPR-Cas9, have revolutionized our ability to study and manipulate mutations. These tools enable scientists to identify mutations responsible for genetic disorders, develop targeted therapies, and improve patient outcomes.

By unraveling the causes and consequences of mutations, we gain a deeper understanding of human health and disease. This knowledge informs medical diagnosis, treatment, and prevention strategies, paving the way for personalized medicine and improved public health outcomes.

# CHAPTER 6: THE ILLUSION OF THE "MAGIC PILL": UNORTHODOX MARKETING AND INCOMPLETE DATA IN DIABETES TREATMENT

The concept of the "magic pill" in the context of treating diabetes often refers to certain medications, such as certain classes of antidiabetic drugs or weight loss medications, that promise rapid weight loss and improved blood sugar control. However, while these medications may offer short-term benefits, they can also come with serious risks and potential drawbacks, including addiction and liver damage.

One example of a medication often marketed as a "magic pill" for weight loss and diabetes treatment is a class of drugs called incretin mimetics, which includes medications like exenatide and liraglutide. These drugs work by mimicking the action of incretin hormones in the body, which help to regulate blood sugar levels. In addition to improving blood sugar control, incretin mimetics have also been associated with weight loss in some individuals. However, these medications can have side effects such as nausea, vomiting, and pancreatitis, and their long-term safety and efficacy for weight loss are still being studied.

Another example is the use of certain weight loss medications, such as phentermine or lorcaserin, in individuals with diabetes or obesity. These medications work by suppressing appetite or reducing the absorption of fat in the body, leading to weight loss. While they may provide short-term benefits in terms of weight loss and blood sugar control, they can also be addictive and have serious side effects, including liver damage, increased heart rate, and psychiatric issues.

It's important to recognize that there is no "magic pill" for managing diabetes or achieving sustainable weight loss. While medications can be an important part of diabetes treatment and weight management for some individuals, they should be used in conjunction with lifestyle changes such as diet modification, regular physical activity, and behavioral therapy. Additionally, the risks and benefits of medication should be carefully weighed, and individuals should work closely with their healthcare providers to develop a comprehensive treatment plan that meets their individual needs and goals.

The concept of the "magic pill" often extends beyond the medication itself to encompass the marketing strategies employed by pharmaceutical companies. In the quest for profit and market dominance, some unscrupulous pharmaceutical companies resort to unorthodox marketing strategies to lure the general public, often without providing complete studies with reliable data samples.

These companies may heavily promote their medications as revolutionary solutions for diabetes and weight loss through aggressive advertising campaigns, celebrity endorsements, and direct-to-consumer marketing tactics. They may exaggerate the benefits of their drugs while downplaying or omitting information about potential risks and side effects.

In the rat race for me-first, some pharmaceutical companies

employ unethical practices, such as selectively publishing favorable study results while withholding unfavorable data or manipulating study designs to produce more favorable outcomes. This cherry-picking of data can create a distorted picture of a medication's safety and efficacy, misleading both healthcare professionals and the general public.

One common scenario is the use of excessively small control groups in clinical trials, which can skew the results and make it difficult to draw accurate conclusions about the safety and efficacy of a medication. When studies are based on small sample sizes, the findings may not be representative of the broader population, leading to inflated claims about the effectiveness of the treatment.

Another problematic practice is failing to blind participants to the treatment they are receiving in clinical trials. Blinding helps to eliminate bias and ensure that participants' expectations do not influence the outcome of the study. When participants are aware of the treatment they are receiving, they may inadvertently alter their behavior or report outcomes differently, leading to biased results.

In both cases, the lack of robust study design and methodology compromises the integrity of the research and calls into question the reliability of the findings. Yet, mass media outlets often report on these studies uncritically, amplifying the pharmaceutical industry's marketing messages and contributing to the proliferation of misinformation.

In their pursuit of profits, these companies may prioritize sales and market share over patient safety, exploiting vulnerable individuals desperate for a quick fix to their health problems. This can lead to a dangerous cycle of overprescribing medications, exposing patients to unnecessary risks and potential harm.

Furthermore, the lack of transparent and comprehensive data can hinder healthcare providers' ability to make informed decisions about medication prescribing and management. Without access to reliable studies with robust data samples, healthcare providers may struggle to accurately assess the risks and benefits of a medication for their patients, potentially compromising patient care.

It is essential for healthcare professionals and consumers alike to critically evaluate the claims and marketing tactics used by pharmaceutical companies and demand transparency, accountability, and rigorous scientific evidence. By advocating for evidence-based medicine and holding pharmaceutical companies accountable for their marketing practices, we can help ensure that patients receive safe and effective treatments that truly benefit their health and well-being.

Ultimately, the pursuit of a "magic pill" for diabetes and weight loss can be risky and potentially harmful. Instead, a holistic approach that addresses the underlying factors contributing to diabetes and obesity, including diet, exercise, and behavioral factors, is essential for long-term success and overall health.

## *Intermezzo*

### WARNING: INSTANT TRANSFORMATION

In an ironic twist, mass media plays a significant role in perpetuating the myth of the "magic pill" for weight loss and diabetes treatment, often without thoroughly investigating clinical studies. Again, pardon the petulance, pharmaceutical companies, driven by profit motives, leverage mass media channels to disseminate their marketing messages, capitalizing on sensationalism and oversimplification to capture the public's attention.

Through glossy advertisements, catchy slogans, and persuasive narratives, these companies paint an enticing picture of their medications as effortless solutions to complex health problems. The promise of rapid weight loss and improved blood sugar control is tantalizing, especially in a society conditioned to seek quick fixes and instant gratification.

However, behind the facade of glamorous marketing lies a darker reality. Many of these medications come with significant risks and potential side effects, which may be downplayed or omitted altogether in mass media campaigns. Furthermore, the evidence supporting the efficacy of these drugs is often incomplete or based on studies with limited sample sizes or short-term follow-up periods.

Despite these shortcomings, mass media outlets often fail to critically examine the validity of pharmaceutical claims or scrutinize the quality of the evidence supporting them. Sensational headlines and clickbait articles grab attention, while nuanced discussions of clinical trial data and scientific methodology are relegated to the sidelines.

Even self-proclaimed prestigious news hubs such as The Financial Times and The Economist are shooting themselves in the foot by proliferating such nonsense. In their pursuit of readership and advertising revenue, they may inadvertently lend credibility to pharmaceutical marketing messages, further perpetuating the illusion of the "magic pill."

As a result, consumers are bombarded with messages promoting the "magic pill" narrative, leading to unrealistic expectations and misplaced trust in pharmaceutical solutions. Patients may be misled into believing that medication alone can solve their health woes, neglecting the importance of lifestyle changes, diet modification, and holistic approaches to disease management.

In this era of information overload, it is more important than ever for consumers to exercise critical thinking and skepticism when evaluating health-related claims. By seeking out reliable sources of information, consulting with healthcare professionals, and advocating for transparency and accountability in pharmaceutical marketing, individuals can empower themselves to make informed decisions about their health and well-being.

*Continuous use of pharmaceutical drugs can indeed have a correlation with liver damage. Here's how:*

1. Drug Metabolism: The liver plays a crucial role in metabolizing drugs. When drugs are ingested, they are broken down by enzymes in the liver, a process known as drug metabolism. Some drugs may produce toxic byproducts during metabolism, which can damage liver cells over time, leading to liver damage or even failure.

2. Drug-Induced Liver Injury (DILI): Certain drugs have been linked to causing liver injury, a condition known as drug-induced liver injury (DILI). This can occur due to various reasons, including direct toxicity of the drug, hypersensitivity reactions, or immune-mediated responses. Chronic use or high doses of medications such as acetaminophen, non-steroidal anti-inflammatory drugs (NSAIDs), statins, and certain antibiotics have been associated with DILI.

3. Chronic Conditions: Patients with chronic health conditions often require long-term medication management. Unfortunately, some of these medications may pose a risk of liver damage over time. For example, individuals with diabetes may take medications such as metformin or thiazolidinediones, which can affect liver function. Similarly, patients with autoimmune diseases may be prescribed immunosuppressant drugs, which can also impact liver health.

4. Drug-Drug Interactions: The liver metabolizes not only prescription drugs but also over-the-counter medications, supplements, and herbs. Taking multiple drugs simultaneously can increase the risk of drug-drug interactions, leading to liver toxicity. This risk is heightened in individuals with pre-existing liver conditions or compromised liver function.

5. Individual Variability: It's essential to recognize that not everyone will experience liver damage from pharmaceutical drugs. Factors such as genetic predisposition, underlying liver disease, age, sex, and concurrent use of other substances (such as alcohol) can influence an individual's susceptibility to drug-

induced liver injury.

Indeed, while pharmaceutical drugs play a vital role in managing various health conditions, it's crucial to be aware of the potential risks they pose to liver health. Patients should work closely with their healthcare providers to monitor liver function regularly, especially when taking medications known to carry a risk of liver damage. Additionally, practicing moderation, avoiding alcohol, and following dosage instructions can help mitigate the risk of liver injury associated with pharmaceutical drug use.

# CHAPTER 7: IGNITING CHANGE: STRATEGIES FOR COMBATTING OBESITY

In a world where the prevalence of obesity continues to rise, it's imperative to ignite change. This chapter delves into innovative strategies aimed at combatting obesity, offering insights into effective approaches for individuals, communities, and policymakers.

1. Empowering Individuals:
   - Education and Awareness: Empowering individuals with knowledge about healthy eating habits, portion control, and the importance of regular physical activity.
   - Behavior Change Techniques: Implementing behavior change techniques, such as goal setting, self-monitoring, and social support networks, to promote sustainable lifestyle modifications.
   - Mindful Eating: Encouraging mindfulness practices to cultivate a healthier relationship with food and prevent overeating.

2. Creating Supportive Environments:
   - Access to Nutritious Foods: Increasing access to affordable, nutritious foods, particularly in underserved communities,

through initiatives such as farmers' markets, community gardens, and healthy food retail programs.

- Built Environment: Designing communities with walkable neighborhoods, bike lanes, and parks to promote physical activity and active transportation.

- Workplace Wellness Programs: Implementing workplace wellness programs that support healthy eating and physical activity among employees, fostering a culture of health and well-being.

3. Policy and Systems Change:

- Sugar Taxes: Advocating for policies such as sugar taxes to reduce the consumption of sugary beverages and incentivize healthier beverage choices.

- Food Labeling: Supporting transparent food labeling initiatives that provide clear information about the nutritional content of packaged foods and beverages.

- School Nutrition Programs: Strengthening school nutrition programs to ensure access to healthy meals and snacks for children, promoting lifelong healthy eating habits.

4. Community Engagement and Advocacy:

- Grassroots Initiatives: Mobilizing community members and organizations to advocate for policies and programs that promote healthy eating and active living.

- Social Marketing Campaigns: Launching social marketing campaigns to raise awareness about the importance of obesity prevention and encourage positive behavior change.

- Coalition Building: Building coalitions and partnerships across sectors, including healthcare, education, government, and business, to address obesity comprehensively and collaboratively.

By igniting change through empowering individuals, creating supportive environments, advocating for policy and systems change, and engaging communities, we can combat the obesity epidemic and create a healthier future for all. It's time to take action and spark meaningful transformation in our communities and society at large.

## Moving from Awareness to Action

While the previous chapter may have seemed straightforward, the issues surrounding obesity are anything but simple. It's true that merely raising awareness is not enough; actionable solutions are essential for meaningful change.

1. Understanding Complexity:
   - Obesity is a multifaceted problem influenced by a myriad of factors, including genetics, environment, culture, and socioeconomic status. Solutions must address these complexities comprehensively rather than oversimplify the issue.
   - Recognizing that individual behavior change is just one piece of the puzzle. Structural changes to environments, policies, and systems are equally crucial for sustainable progress.

2. Shifting Perspectives:
   - Emphasizing the importance of shifting societal attitudes and norms surrounding body image, weight, and health. Promoting acceptance, inclusivity, and respect for diverse body shapes and sizes can help reduce stigma and improve mental well-being.
   - Encouraging a shift from a focus on weight loss to a broader emphasis on overall health and well-being. This includes promoting balanced nutrition, regular physical activity, and positive body image.

3. Advocating for Equity:
   - Acknowledging the disproportionate burden of obesity borne by marginalized communities, including racial and ethnic minorities, low-income populations, and individuals with disabilities. Solutions must prioritize equity and address underlying social determinants of health.
   - Advocating for policies and interventions that promote

health equity and address systemic inequalities in access to resources, opportunities, and healthcare services.

4. Fostering Collaboration:
   - Highlighting the importance of collaboration across sectors and disciplines to address obesity comprehensively. This includes engaging healthcare providers, policymakers, educators, community leaders, and individuals affected by obesity in collaborative efforts.
   - Facilitating dialogue and knowledge-sharing between stakeholders to identify innovative solutions, leverage resources, and maximize impact. By working together, we can amplify our collective efforts and drive meaningful change.

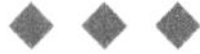

While the challenges of combatting obesity may seem daunting, they are not insurmountable. By embracing complexity, shifting perspectives, advocating for equity, and fostering collaboration, we can move beyond awareness to action. Let's embark on this journey together, with a commitment to creating a healthier, more equitable future for all.

# REFERENCES


- Bleich, S. N., et al. (2020). Effects of beverage taxes on purchases and dietary intake: A systematic review and meta-analysis. American Journal of Public Health, 110(3), e1-e8.
- Centers for Disease Control and Prevention. (2020). Strategies to prevent obesity and other chronic diseases: The CDC guide to strategies to increase the consumption of fruits and vegetables. CDC.
- Evans, W. D., et al. (2015). Systematic review and meta-analysis of the effectiveness of mass media interventions for child survival in low- and middle-income countries. Journal of Health Communication, 20(S1), 11-23.
- Greaves, C. J., et al. (2011). Systematic review of reviews of intervention components associated with increased effectiveness in dietary and physical activity interventions. BMC Public Health, 11(1), 119.
- Katterman, S. N., et al. (2014). Mindfulness meditation as an intervention for binge eating, emotional eating, and weight loss: A systematic review. Eating Behaviors, 15(2), 197-204.
- Khan, L. K., et al. (2017). Recommended community strategies and measurements to prevent obesity in the United States. MMWR Recommendations and Reports, 66(6), 1-26.
- Kumanyika, S. K., et al. (2009). Community energy balance: A framework for contextualizing cultural influences on high risk of obesity in ethnic minority populations. Preventive Medicine, 49(5), 345-353.
- Matson-Koffman, D. M., et al. (2005). Evidence-based interventions to promote physical activity: What contributes to

dissemination by state health departments. American Journal of Preventive Medicine, 29(1), 73-80.

*Building a Healthier Future:*
*Spreading Awareness and*
*Advocating for Change*

In our modern world, where convenience often trumps health, building a healthier future requires more than just individual efforts. It demands collective action, awareness, and advocacy. This chapter explores the vital role of spreading awareness and advocating for change in combatting the obesity epidemic and fostering a culture of wellness.

## The Power Of Awareness

Spreading awareness is the first step towards addressing any public health issue, and obesity is no exception. By educating individuals about the risks of obesity, the importance of healthy lifestyle choices, and the societal factors contributing to the epidemic, we can empower them to make informed decisions about their health. Awareness campaigns can take many forms, from public service announcements and educational materials to social media campaigns and community events. These initiatives aim to reach people where they are, leveraging various channels to disseminate information and spark conversations about obesity prevention and management.

## Advocating For Change

Awareness alone is not enough to drive meaningful change; advocacy is essential to translate awareness into action. Advocacy involves speaking out, raising concerns, and mobilizing support for policies and programs that promote healthy environments and behaviors. This may include advocating for legislation to regulate the marketing of unhealthy foods and beverages, improve access to nutritious foods in underserved communities, or implement school-based nutrition and physical activity initiatives. Advocates play a crucial role in amplifying the voices of those affected by obesity, holding policymakers and stakeholders accountable, and championing evidence-based solutions to address the root causes of the epidemic.

## Collaborative Efforts

Building a healthier future requires collaboration across sectors and disciplines. Governments, healthcare providers, educators, businesses, community organizations, and individuals all have a role to play in addressing obesity comprehensively. Collaborative efforts bring together diverse perspectives, resources, and expertise to develop and implement multifaceted strategies that tackle the complex drivers of the epidemic. By working together towards a common goal, we can leverage our collective strengths and make a greater impact on population health and well-being.

## Inspiring Action

Ultimately, building a healthier future is about inspiring action at all levels of society. Whether it's advocating for policy changes, supporting community-based initiatives, or making healthier choices in our daily lives, each of us has the power to contribute to positive change. By raising awareness, advocating for change, and collaborating with others, we can create environments that support healthy choices, empower individuals to lead healthier lives, and build a future where obesity is no longer a widespread public health concern.

Let us join forces, raise our voices, and take action together to build a healthier future for ourselves, our communities, and future generations. The time for change is now, and together, we can make it happen.

# CHAPTER 8: MINDFUL INDULGENCE: FINDING BALANCE IN A WORLD OF EXCESS

In a society that often encourages overconsumption and indulgence, the practice of mindfulness offers a powerful antidote. Mindfulness, rooted in ancient contemplative traditions, invites us to cultivate present-moment awareness and non-judgmental acceptance of our thoughts, feelings, and sensations. By bringing mindful attention to our eating habits and behaviors, we can develop a deeper understanding of our relationship with food and make more conscious choices that support our health and well-being.

## Exploring Mindful Eating

Mindful eating is a practice that encourages us to slow down and savor each bite, engaging all of our senses in the experience of eating. By paying close attention to the taste, texture, and aroma of our food, we can enhance our enjoyment and satisfaction while also becoming more attuned to our body's hunger and fullness cues. Mindful eating allows us to savor the flavors of our meals without the need for excessive quantities, fostering a greater sense of gratitude and contentment with what we have.

# Navigating Temptation With Awareness

In a world filled with tempting treats and indulgent delights, mindfulness can serve as a valuable tool for navigating moments of temptation. By bringing awareness to our cravings and impulses, we can observe them without immediately acting on them, allowing space for reflection and discernment. Mindfulness invites us to inquire into the underlying causes of our desires, whether they arise from genuine hunger, emotional needs, or societal influences, empowering us to make choices that align with our values and intentions.

# Cultivating Self-Compassion

Practicing mindfulness also involves cultivating self-compassion and kindness towards ourselves, especially in moments of perceived failure or indulgence. Instead of berating ourselves for giving in to cravings or overeating, we can approach ourselves with understanding and forgiveness, recognizing that we are human and imperfect. Through self-compassion, we can learn from our experiences without judgment, fostering a sense of inner resilience and self-worth that transcends external measures of success or failure.

# Building Resilience Against Overindulgence

Mindfulness empowers us to develop greater resilience against the allure of overindulgence by fostering a deeper connection to our inner wisdom and values. By tuning into our body's signals and honoring its needs with care and respect, we can cultivate a more balanced and harmonious relationship with food. Mindfulness also encourages us to explore alternative sources of pleasure and fulfillment beyond material indulgence, such as cultivating meaningful relationships, engaging in creative pursuits, and connecting with nature.

## Embracing Mindful Living

In a culture that often equates happiness with consumption and excess, the practice of mindfulness offers a path towards a more meaningful and fulfilling way of life. By cultivating present-moment awareness, self-compassion, and resilience, we can navigate the complexities of modern living with greater wisdom and grace. Through mindful eating and mindful living, we can find balance and contentment in a world of abundance, embracing each moment with gratitude and awareness.

# CHAPTER 9: ODDITY AT PLAY

Here's a sad story that serves as a terrible wake-up call. In Dallas, Texas, there stands a notorious restaurant with a bold sign that dares tourists to enter, warning them of the potential lethality of its offerings. The most recent casualty of its indulgent menu was Glenn River, alias, a mere twenty-nine years old, who had unwittingly become the face of the establishment, even gracing television commercials. At a staggering two hundred and seventy pounds, he embodied the stark consequences of succumbing to the allure of the restaurant's fare.

When pressed about his culpability in the tragic demise of one of his regular patrons, the restaurant owner's response was as cold as it was calculated:

"Absolutely! It's all good publicity for my joint. Those who revile me end up inadvertently promoting my restaurant in the press, making it a must-visit attraction for tourists. Where else can you feast on an eight-patty, eight-thousand-calorie monstrosity? Sure, I might be contributing to people's demise, but so are all those other eateries peddling this junk food."

While this tale may sound like satire, it offers a stark glimpse into the culture of excess, deceptive advertising, and widespread obesity that plagues not just Dallas, but the entirety of the United States. The brazen acknowledgment of the inherent dangers of the food served reflects a disturbing lack of regulation or concern for food quality in certain corners of the industry. Glenn River's tragic end serves as a sobering reminder of the real risks associated with excessive consumption of unhealthy fare.

The owner's cynical and unapologetic response to the loss of a loyal customer lays bare the distorted priorities rampant in American food culture, where profit often takes precedence over consumer well-being. His callous belief that "any publicity is good publicity" is emblematic of the mercenary mindset that too often drives decision-making in the food industry.

In the wake of Glenn River's passing, the government's declaration of war on obesity may seem like a justified response to a burgeoning public health crisis. However, the introduction of "tour de force camps" as a solution to weight loss raises questions about the ethics of an industry that profits from exploiting people's health problems. The exorbitant cost of these programs underscores the stark reality of limited access to resources for addressing obesity, highlighting the pervasive socioeconomic inequalities that influence individuals' health outcomes.

Lastly, the rhetorical question, "What's in it for me?" serves as a poignant reflection of the prevailing individualistic ethos that pervades American society, where personal gain often outweighs considerations of social responsibility or the common good.

## Interpretation

In the aftermath of Glenn River's tragic death, both the local and national communities were rocked by shock and disbelief. News outlets rushed to cover the story, with headlines ranging from sensationalist exposes to somber reflections on the state of American health. Social media platforms buzzed with speculation, outrage, and calls for action, as individuals grappled with the sobering reality of one man's demise at the hands of his own dietary choices.

Locally, in Dallas, the restaurant at the center of the controversy found itself thrust into the spotlight. Once bustling dining rooms now sat eerily quiet as patrons wrestled with the implications of Glenn's passing. While some loyal customers remained steadfast in their support, dismissing the tragedy as an isolated incident or even defending the restaurant's right to serve whatever fare it pleased, others recoiled in horror. Some vowed never to set foot in the establishment again, calling for its immediate closure.

Nationally, Glenn River's death sparked a broader conversation about the pervasive issue of obesity in America. Experts weighed in on the root causes of the epidemic, pointing fingers at sedentary lifestyles, poor dietary choices, systemic inequalities, and the influence of the food industry. Advocacy groups seized upon the tragedy as a rallying cry, renewing their calls for stricter regulations on food advertising, improved access to healthy foods in underserved communities, and greater investment in public health initiatives.

In the midst of the media frenzy and public outcry, Glenn River's family found themselves thrust into the spotlight. Their grief was laid bare for the world to see. While some sought solace in private mourning, others chose to speak out, sharing their son's story in the hope of preventing similar tragedies from befalling others. Their courage and resilience in the face of unimaginable loss served as a powerful reminder of the human toll of the obesity epidemic and the urgent need for meaningful change.

As the dust settled and the news cycle moved on to the next headline, the question remained: what would society do with this wake-up call? Would we continue down the path of least resistance, content to turn a blind eye to the consequences of our collective indulgence? Or would we seize this opportunity to confront the uncomfortable truths about our relationship with food and take meaningful steps towards building a healthier, more equitable future for all? The choice, ultimately, is ours to make.

# CHAPTER 10: CONCLUSION: OUR COLLECTIVE RESPONSIBILITY TO COMBAT OBESITY

As we reach the end of this journey, it's essential to recognize that combatting obesity is not solely an individual endeavor—it's a collective responsibility that requires action from all levels of society. Each of us plays a crucial role in addressing this epidemic and building a healthier future for ourselves and generations to come.

From policymakers shaping public health policies to healthcare providers offering guidance and support, from educators instilling healthy habits in our youth to businesses promoting nutritious options, we all have a part to play. But our responsibilities don't end there. As individuals, we must take ownership of our health, making informed choices and advocating for change in our communities.

It's time to break the cycle of inactivity and unhealthy eating habits, to challenge the status quo, and to create environments that support health and well-being. It won't be easy, and it won't happen overnight, but together, we can make a difference.

Let's commit to spreading awareness, advocating for change,

and supporting one another on this journey towards a healthier future. By working together, we can overcome the challenges of obesity and create a world where everyone has the opportunity to thrive.

The time for action is now. Let's stand together and embrace our collective responsibility to combat obesity, paving the way for a brighter, healthier tomorrow. Thanks for reading.

## Suggested actions

Individuals have the power to make informed choices about their diet and lifestyle. By prioritizing healthy eating habits, regular physical activity, and adequate sleep, individuals can take control of their health and reduce their risk of obesity. Seeking professional guidance from healthcare providers and registered dietitians can further support individuals in their journey towards a healthier weight.

Families and communities play a vital role in shaping attitudes and behaviors around food and physical activity. Creating supportive environments that encourage healthy choices and provide access to nutritious food and safe spaces for physical activity is essential. Schools, workplaces, and community organizations can implement programs and policies that promote healthy lifestyles and empower individuals to make positive changes.

The food industry has a significant responsibility to reformulate products, reduce portion sizes, and limit marketing of unhealthy foods, particularly to children. Transparent labeling and responsible advertising practices are crucial to empower consumers to make informed choices.

Governments and policymakers must prioritize obesity prevention and implement comprehensive strategies that address the various factors contributing to the epidemic. This includes enacting policies that promote healthy food environments, support physical activity infrastructure, and invest in public health education and awareness campaigns.

Healthcare professionals play a critical role in identifying and managing obesity. By providing compassionate, evidence-based care and promoting preventative measures, healthcare providers can empower patients to take charge of their health and reduce their risk of obesity-related complications.

Combating obesity requires a multi-pronged approach that addresses individual behaviors, environmental factors, and systemic issues. By acknowledging our collective responsibility and working collaboratively across sectors, we can create a future where healthy choices are accessible and supported, ultimately leading to a healthier population and a reduction in the burden of obesity.

# GLOSSARY

1. Obesity: A medical condition characterized by excess body fat accumulation, often resulting in adverse health effects such as cardiovascular disease, diabetes, and certain cancers.

2. BMI (Body Mass Index): A measure of body fat based on height and weight, commonly used to classify individuals as underweight, normal weight, overweight, or obese.

3. Fast Food: Convenient, mass-produced food that is typically high in calories, fat, sugar, and salt, and low in nutritional value. Often associated with the rise of obesity due to its affordability, accessibility, and palatability.

4. Fat Tax: A proposed tax on foods and beverages high in calories, fat, sugar, or salt, intended to discourage consumption and generate revenue to offset the societal costs of obesity-related health problems.

5. Sedentary Lifestyle: A lifestyle characterized by little to no physical activity, often associated with increased risk of obesity and related health issues.

6. Nutritional Education: Programs aimed at teaching individuals about healthy eating habits, portion control, and the importance of a balanced diet in maintaining overall health and preventing obesity.

7. Food Industry: The sector of the economy involved in the production, processing, distribution, and marketing of food and beverages, which plays a significant role in shaping dietary habits

and contributing to the obesity epidemic.

8. Public Health Initiatives: Government-led efforts to promote and protect the health of populations through measures such as health education, disease prevention, and access to healthcare services, with a focus on addressing the root causes of obesity.

9. Body Positivity: A social movement advocating for acceptance and appreciation of all body types, challenging societal norms and stereotypes surrounding beauty and health, and promoting self-love and confidence regardless of size.

10. Fitness Industry: The sector of the economy involved in providing products and services related to physical fitness and exercise, including gyms, personal trainers, fitness equipment, and wellness programs.

11. Food Deserts: Geographic areas with limited access to affordable, nutritious food options, often due to socioeconomic factors such as poverty, lack of transportation, and the concentration of fast food outlets.

12. Nutrient Density: The ratio of nutrients (such as vitamins, minerals, and fiber) to calories in a food or beverage, with higher nutrient density indicating a greater concentration of essential nutrients relative to energy content.

13. Portion Control: The practice of moderating food and beverage intake to ensure appropriate serving sizes, often used as a strategy for managing weight and preventing overconsumption.

14. Health Disparities: Differences in health outcomes and access to healthcare services experienced by individuals or communities based on factors such as race, ethnicity, socioeconomic status, geography, and education level.

15. Health Literacy: The ability to obtain, understand, and use information and services to make informed decisions about health, including navigating healthcare systems, interpreting

medical advice, and accessing appropriate resources for prevention and treatment.

# SUGGESTED READINGS

1. "Mindful Eating: A Guide to Rediscovering a Healthy and Joyful Relationship with Food" by Jan Chozen Bays

- This book offers practical guidance and exercises for incorporating mindfulness into your eating habits, helping you develop a more mindful and intuitive approach to food.

2. "The Mindful Diet: How to Transform Your Relationship with Food for Lasting Weight Loss and Vibrant Health" by Ruth Wolever and Beth Reardon

- Combining mindfulness practices with evidence-based nutrition strategies, this book provides a comprehensive framework for achieving sustainable weight loss and improved well-being.

3. "Savor: Mindful Eating, Mindful Life" by Thich Nhat Hanh and Lilian Cheung

- Written by renowned mindfulness teacher Thich Nhat Hanh and nutritionist Lilian Cheung, this book explores the connection between mindfulness and eating, offering practical exercises and meditations to cultivate mindful awareness in everyday life.

4. "The Obesity Code: Unlocking the Secrets of Weight Loss" by Dr. Jason Fung

- Dr. Jason Fung presents a compelling argument against conventional wisdom on obesity, exploring the role of insulin resistance and metabolic dysfunction in weight gain. This book offers practical strategies for addressing the root causes of obesity and achieving sustainable weight loss.

5. "In Defense of Food: An Eater's Manifesto" by Michael Pollan
- Michael Pollan examines the modern Western diet and its impact on health, advocating for a return to simple, whole foods and mindful eating practices. This book offers valuable insights into the cultural and environmental factors influencing our food choices.

6. "The Joy of Half a Cookie: Using Mindfulness to Lose Weight and End the Struggle with Food" by Jean Kristeller
- Dr. Jean Kristeller, a leading researcher in the field of mindfulness-based eating awareness training (MB-EAT), shares practical strategies for using mindfulness to overcome emotional eating and develop a healthier relationship with food.

7. "Eating Mindfully: How to End Mindless Eating and Enjoy a Balanced Relationship with Food" by Susan Albers
- Dr. Susan Albers offers a step-by-step guide to practicing mindful eating, with exercises, meditations, and self-reflection prompts to help readers develop greater awareness and appreciation for the food they eat.

8. "Salt Sugar Fat: How the Food Giants Hooked Us" by Michael Moss
- Investigative journalist Michael Moss exposes the tactics used by the food industry to manipulate consumer behavior and promote overconsumption of processed foods high in salt, sugar, and fat. This book sheds light on the societal factors contributing to the obesity epidemic and the need for systemic change.

These books provide valuable insights and practical tools for anyone interested in exploring the intersection of mindfulness, healthy eating, and combating obesity. Whether you're looking to deepen your understanding of mindful living or seeking strategies for improving your relationship with food, these readings offer valuable resources for your journey toward greater health and well-being.

# BOOKS BY THIS AUTHOR

## Excellence Won't Save You

In a world obsessed with the pursuit of excellence, where success is often equated with perfection, it's time to challenge the status quo. "Excellence Won't Save You" invites readers on a thought-provoking journey through the complexities of achievement and the pitfalls of conventional wisdom.

Delving into the depths of history, philosophy, and human psychology, this book unravels the illusions of success that have long captivated our collective consciousness. From the fallacy of reasoning by analogy to the dangers of social media-driven expectations, it sheds light on the myths and misconceptions that surround the pursuit of excellence.

Drawing on real-life examples, captivating narratives, and insightful analysis, "Excellence Won't Save You" offers a fresh perspective on what it truly means to thrive in a world that often values appearances over authenticity. It challenges readers to question their assumptions, embrace uncertainty, and redefine their notions of success.

You'll discover:

The fallacy of reasoning by analogy: Why past achievements don't guarantee future success.
The paradox of excellence: How the relentless pursuit of perfection can lead to disillusionment and burnout.

The importance of authenticity: Why embracing your flaws and vulnerabilities is essential for true fulfillment.
Strategies for resilience: How to navigate failure, setbacks, and uncertainty with grace and resilience.
Redefining success: Why success is more than just external validation or societal expectations.

Whether you're a seasoned leader, a budding entrepreneur, or simply someone searching for meaning in a chaotic world, this book provides a roadmap for navigating the complexities of achievement with clarity and purpose. It's a reminder that true excellence isn't found in perfection, but in the courage to embrace our imperfections and pursue a path that is uniquely our own.

"Excellence Won't Save You" is not just another self-help book—it's a manifesto for those who dare to challenge the status quo, defy the odds, and chart their own course towards a life of meaning and fulfillment. It's time to break free from the illusions of success and discover what truly matters in the pursuit of excellence.

## Asking Good Questions: Unleashing Curiosity For Personal And Professional Growth

Step into a world where questions reign supreme, where curiosity is the driving force behind remarkable achievements. Welcome to the transformative realm of "Asking Good Questions," a captivating book that unveils the secrets to unlocking your full potential through the art of inquiry.

Embark on a captivating journey as you delve into the importance of asking good questions in every facet of your life. From the moment you crack open this compelling guide, you'll be transported into a world where clarity, relevance, and open-endedness become your guiding principles.

Immerse yourself in the sheer power of thought-provoking questions that challenge the status quo and propel you towards innovative thinking. Discover how contextual questioning can breathe life into your conversations, allowing you to navigate diverse situations with ease and finesse.

Explore the art of follow-up and active listening, honing your skills to build meaningful connections and extract deeper insights from those around you. Witness firsthand how different types of questions unlock doors to personal growth, forge stronger relationships, and drive success in business and leadership.

As you journey through the pages of "Asking Good Questions," you'll encounter invaluable tips, practical advice, and actionable strategies that enhance your questioning skills. Whether you're a student, a professional, or an aspiring leader, this book provides the roadmap to sharpening your ability to inquire, challenge, and explore.

With clarity and precision, this work tackles the common obstacles that may impede your questioning prowess. Learn how to overcome them and unleash your curiosity, tapping into a wellspring of inspiration and knowledge that will fuel your personal and professional growth.

## Dear Seeker Of Light: Illuminating The Path To Self-Awareness And Self-Regulation

Let this sacred letter be your compass, guiding you towards the radiant essence of your true self. Realize the transformative power of self-discovery, self-compassion, and resilience as you embrace your authentic path.

"Dear Seeker of Light" is a soul-stirring guide, crafted with love and purpose. It offers solace to weary hearts, and empowers you to live a life infused with meaning, joy, and profound fulfillment.

Embrace the invitation to awaken the dormant seeker within you. Allow the wisdom, warmth, and encouragement to envelop your journey as you navigate the transformative possibilities that lie ahead.